The Smart Life Series
Preventing ACL Injuries in Female Athletes

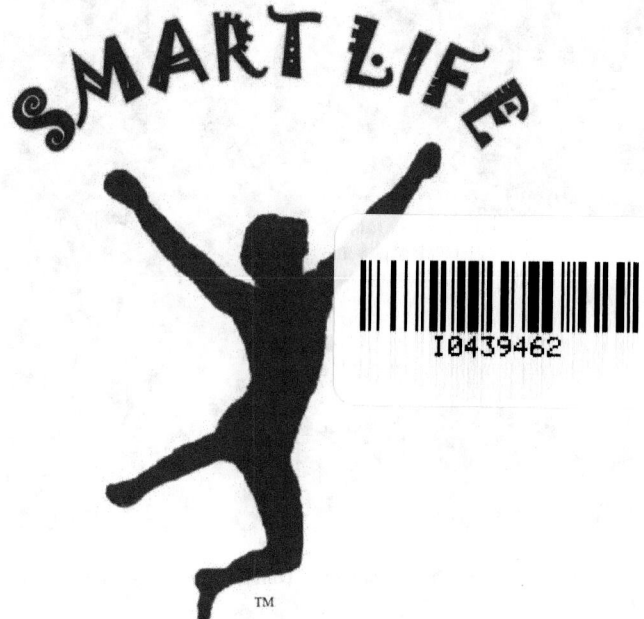

Sean Simonds, PT, DPT, OCS, CSCS

Board Certified Orthopedic Clinical Specialist

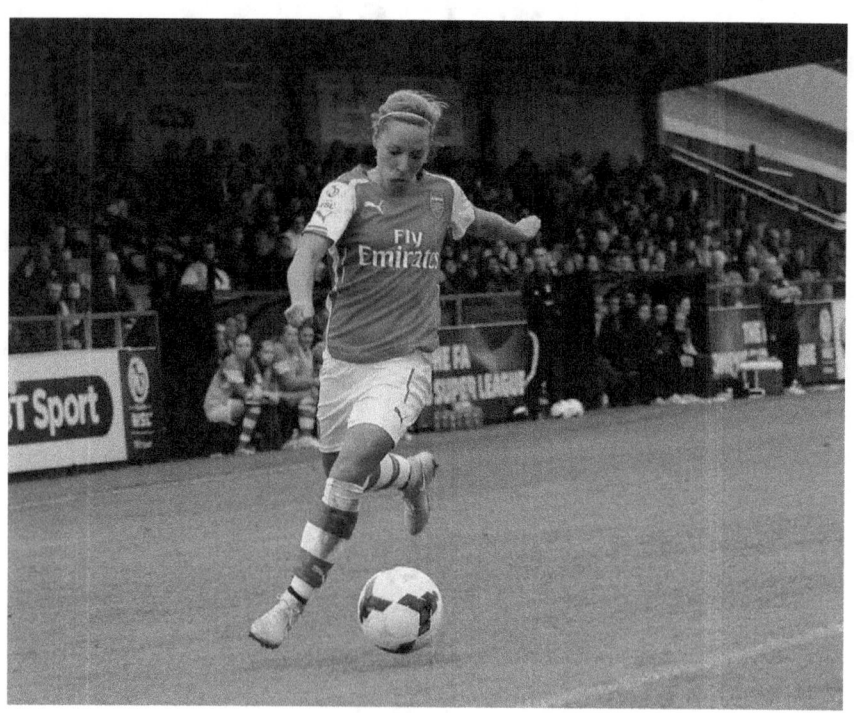

Creative Commons License: http://www.flickr.com/photos/109430286@N06/16280085627

ISBN: 1497494028
ISBN-13: 978-1497494022

DEDICATION

To my loving wife and wonderful family.

CONTENTS

ACKNOWLEDGMENTS

Thanks to my wonderful family for pushing me to create more and do more

What's The Problem?

Why a book about preventing ACL (Anterior Cruciate Ligament of the knee) injuries? ACL injuries are all too common in young athletes. Over 200,000 ACL tears occur in the United States each year. Female athletes are 4-8 times more likely to suffer an ACL injury than males participating in the same sport[1]. Female athletes between the ages of 15 and 20 appear to be at the greatest risk[1]. Adams et al[2] reported that one in every 100 female high school athletes and one in every 10 female college athletes will suffer an ACL injury. ACL injuries are practically an epidemic in female athletes!

But what is the big deal about an ACL injury? Firstly, the injury is quite painful. The biggest problem, however, is that the ACL is a major stabilizing ligament of the knee and so when the ligament is injured it leaves the knee potentially unstable. If the knee joint is left too mobile- it shifts when subjected to strain, as is the case in sports-related movements. This results in pain and leaves the knee dysfunctional and more prone to further injury. When an athlete sustains an ACL tear, it is unlikely she will be able to return to the same level of athletics without repair.

Repair of a torn ACL requires surgery. Surgery and rehabilitation take a lot of time, and is very expensive. Even with surgery, the athlete is out of their sport for many months. In surgery, grafts from a cadaver, or the patient's own tissue, are used to replace the torn ligament. The surgery is usually performed through a TV scope (arthroscope). Total cost of repair can run in the tens of thousands of dollars.

Often the athlete will undergo Physical Therapy both before and after surgery. After surgery, therapy starts in one to two days. Athletes then work intensely with therapists weekly and exercise extensively at home. Initially, they are very restricted in various activities and motions. Athletes may return to light jogging no earlier than 12 weeks after surgery. They may resume some athletics no earlier than 6 months. Generally it takes anywhere from 9 to 18 months to return to full competitive athletics. Confidence and strength have been shown to be a problem in many athletes even after very successful surgery. Many athletes never return to their previous peak athletic performance.

Clearly then, ACL injuries can have a severe impact on the life of an athlete- both physically and emotionally. Prevention of the injury should therefore be paramount to all athletes- particularly female athletes.

Interestingly, most ACL injuries do not occur from contact. 70% occur when the athlete is running hard, cutting, jumping, or twisting[3]. No contact is incurred. Why does this matter? It means that unlucky or freak collisions are **NOT** the cause of most ACL injuries. Rather, the injuries have to do with the condition of the athletes knee versus the stress the athlete puts upon it. A high functioning knee is less likely to be injured with the sudden twists and turns of athletic competition, a poorly conditioned knee is much more prone. Thus, with proper identification of knees that are at risk and subsequent strengthening and conditioning, we can significantly reduce the number of ACL injuries in sports! This is particularly important in female athletes who are so prone to the injury.

That is what this short book is all about- trying to prevent this devastating injury in our female athletes. The full range of knee strength and conditioning exercises is beyond the scope of the book, and should be guided by sports or orthopedic specialty-Physical Therapists (although we will cover some basics). What this book will focus on is how to identify the athlete at risk of the injury, specifically the female athlete[3,4]. The tests outlined in the book are simple and are supplemented by videos on our website (www.youtube.com/TheSmartLifeSeries), so all female athletes should be evaluated. An ounce of prevention is worth a pound of cure, so please read on!

This book is oriented to the athlete herself, coaches, trainers, and even parents. All can be actively involved in assuring the best possible function and health of the athlete's knees.

Please note: ACL risk assessment should be conducted periodically throughout an athlete's career. This is particularly true for athletes who required ACL protection programs due to abnormal mechanics. Such a program only works if the athlete is vigilant about maintenance exercises throughout her athletic career.

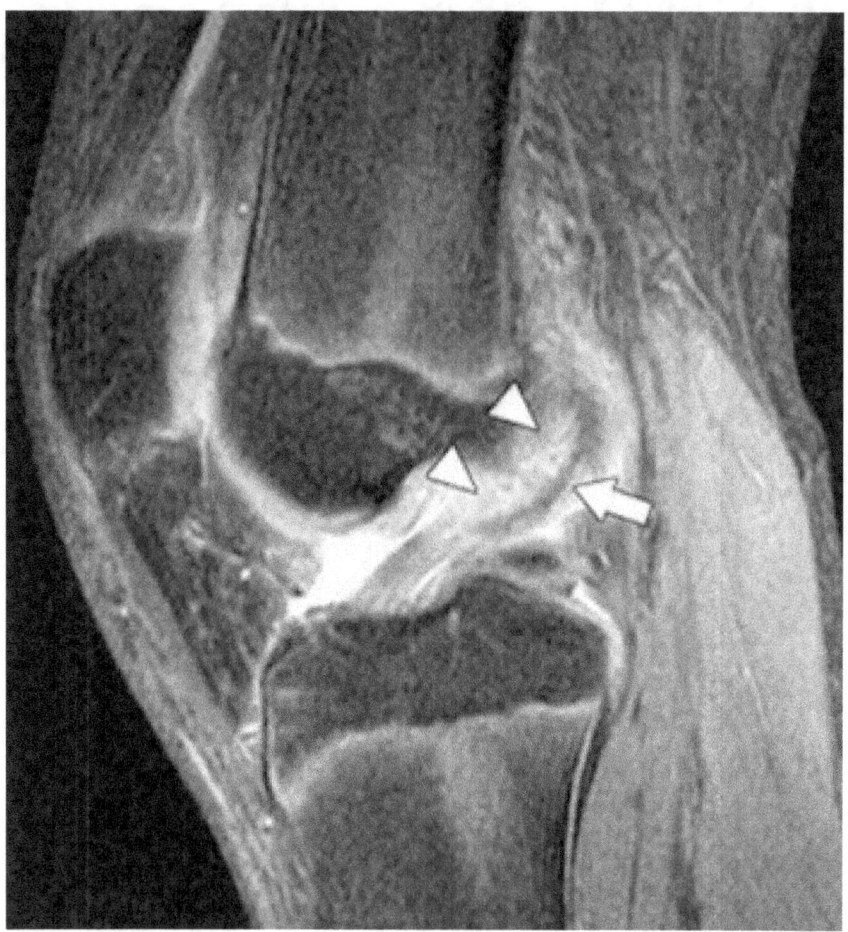

*Thanks to one of my patients for allowing me to include this image.

What Is The ACL?

The ACL is a thick band of tissue that attaches to the two major bones that make up the knee joint. It is a major stabilizer of the knee. The ACL is responsible for limiting the amount of forward motion of the tibia (lower leg) on the femur (thigh bone). It will also restrict the lower leg turning in on the thigh (pictured below). The ACL is identified below along with a couple other major structures.

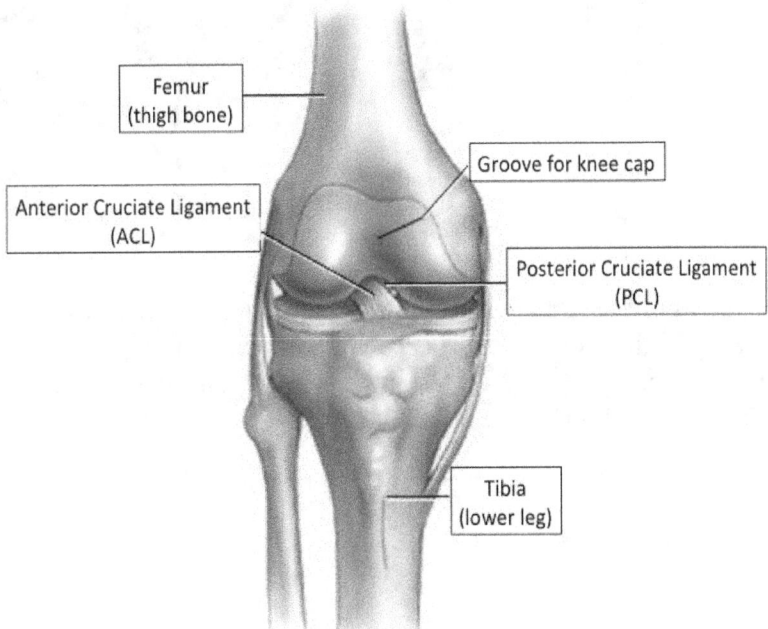

Imagine then, how important this ligament is during a sporting event. Athletes run, jump, twist, cut and change direction constantly in competitions. We need a functioning ACL along with strong muscular support to participate at our body's maximum potential.

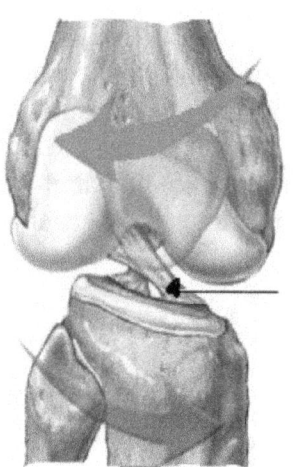 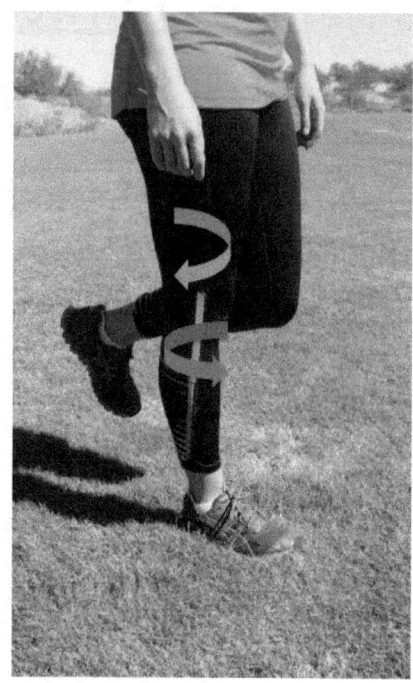

Without a healthy ACL, there is excess movement in the knee making high-intensity exercise and sports challenging, if not impossible. A damaged ACL increases the risk of early-onset arthritis and meniscus tears.

How Do I Know If I'm At Risk For An ACL Injury?

A short but effective assessment of ACL injury risk involves having the athlete squat, hop, lunge, and jog under controlled circumstances. Please note that these are *not* tests to assess whether the ACL is *already torn*. Rather, these are tests to see if the ACL *is at risk* for being torn.

The following 4 activities can easily be performed on any level surface. Many of those at risk for ACL injury can be very easy to spot if you know what to look for. An athlete who demonstrates findings that indicate an increased risk for ACL injury should be sent to a Physical Therapist with a Board Specialty in Orthopedics or Sports for further evaluation and recommendations. Ideally the therapist will coordinate with the athlete's coaches and trainers to optimize their conditioning and lower their risk of injury.

Importantly, it is critical to perform these assessments BEFORE and AFTER a workout/practice. Disposition towards ACL injury may become more evident when the athlete is fatigued. Have the athlete perform 3 sets of 10 repetitions. If you notice any reps that look bad, it is time to send them to a qualified Physical Therapist!

Videos of the following assessments can be found at: www.youtube.com/TheSmartLifeSeries Click on the "**Playlist**" tab and select "**ACL Injury Risk Assessment**."

<u>Squat Assessment</u>

The first function to test is the performance of the knee in a squat. The squat needs to be performed properly to make the knee assessment more valid.

The picture on the following page shows the proper form for a squat (please refer to our videos for more instruction).

1. The hips/knees/and ankles should be lined up from start to finish.
2. The feet should stay flat and pointed forward.
3. The knees should remain shoulder width apart.
4. Weight should be evenly distributed to both legs and the trunk should not lean to either side.
5. Start in the standing position with feet shoulder width apart (see arrows).
6. Hands can be resting at the hips or held at the side.
7. Slowly sit back as if you are sitting in a chair.
8. The squat should be initiated with the hips and should move downwards and backwards.
9. No part of the lower extremities should move forward during this motion.
10. Keep the trunk straight. Only bend at the hips and knees.
11. The hands can come forward to assist with balance.
12. The head should be kept up looking forward throughout the motion.

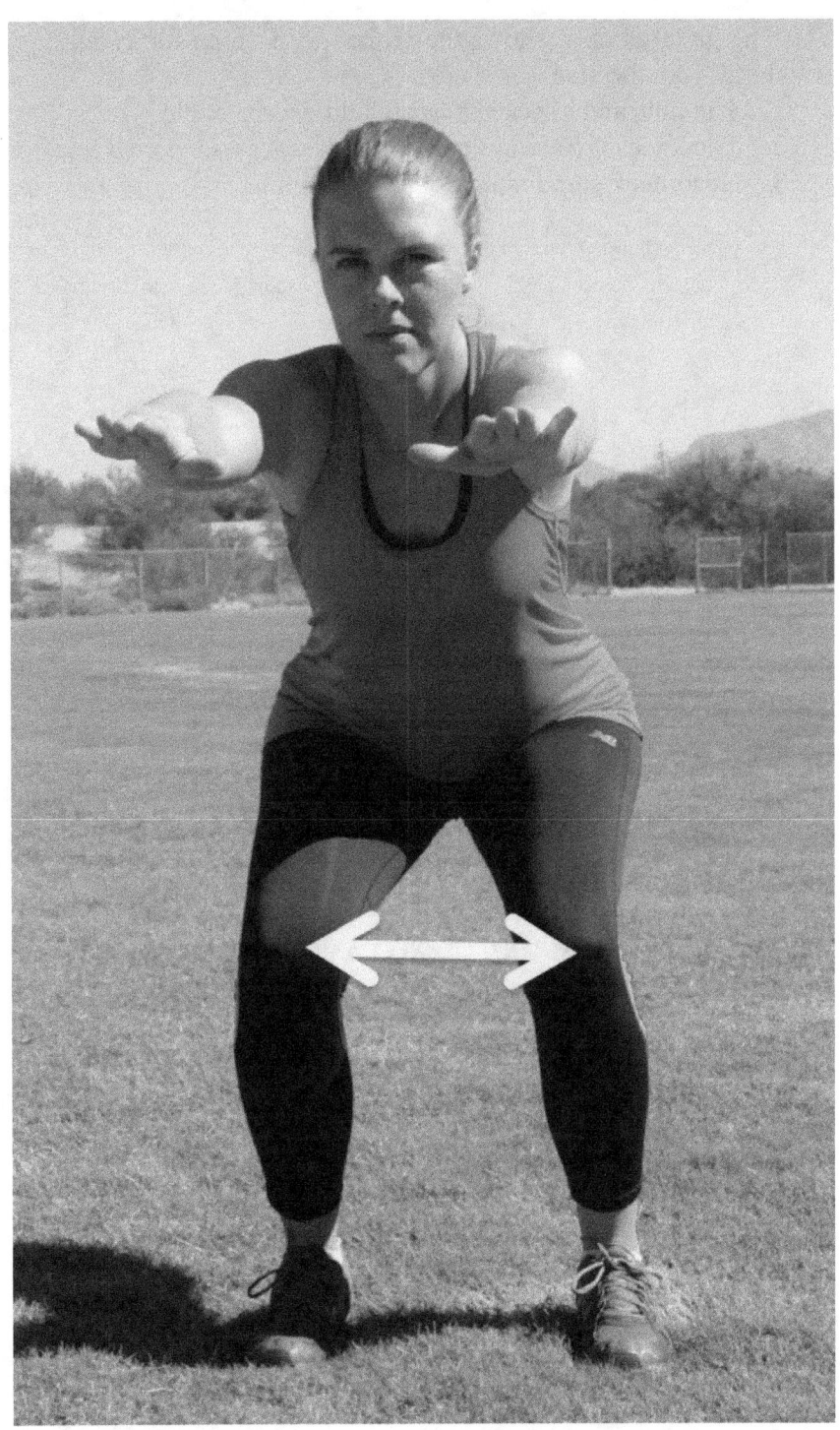

The picture below shows the proper positioning for a squat watching from the side.
1. The hips and knees approach a 90 degree angle.
2. The knees are always be behind the toes (see dotted line).
3. Head/neck/spine maintain a straight line.

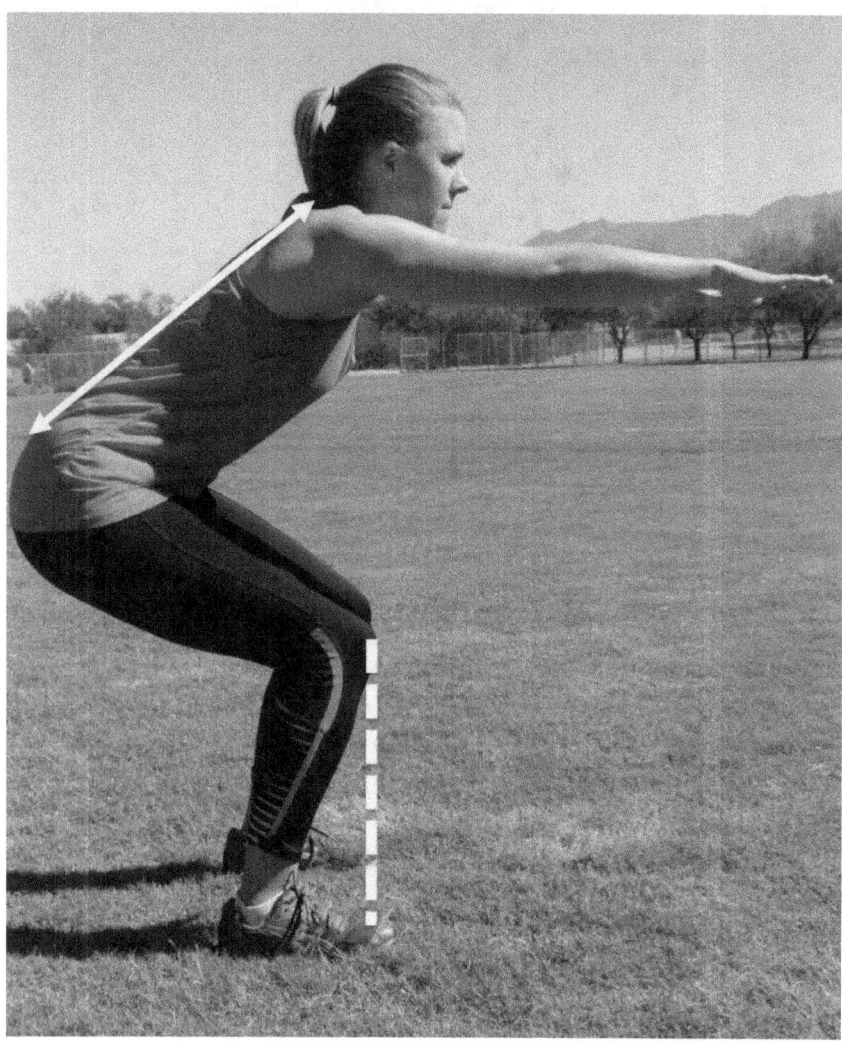

<u>Abnormal Findings on Squat Assessment</u>

    The picture on the next page shows someone *trying* to squat but exhibiting abnormal mechanics and knee dynamics.

1. Note how the knees turn in so that the knee caps are almost facing each other. This is the first sign that the athlete is at risk for an ACL tear. This is often the easiest sign to spot. Try getting into this position (it makes my knees uncomfortable) and then try running with the knees turned in, it hurts! This is an ACL tear just waiting to happen.
2. If the knees dives in towards the middle during running, jumping, squatting, or any other time, this warrants an immediate referral to Physical Therapy!
3. Note how the knees get closer with progression of the squat to the point of almost touching.
4. During the squat, look for a lean in the trunk. If the athlete is leaning to one side this could signal weakness, poor balance, pain, or other conditions that may require evaluation.
5. Also look to see that the athlete keeps her head up at all times. If the athlete looks at the ground this could represent balance problems which are thought to predispose athlete's to ACL injury.

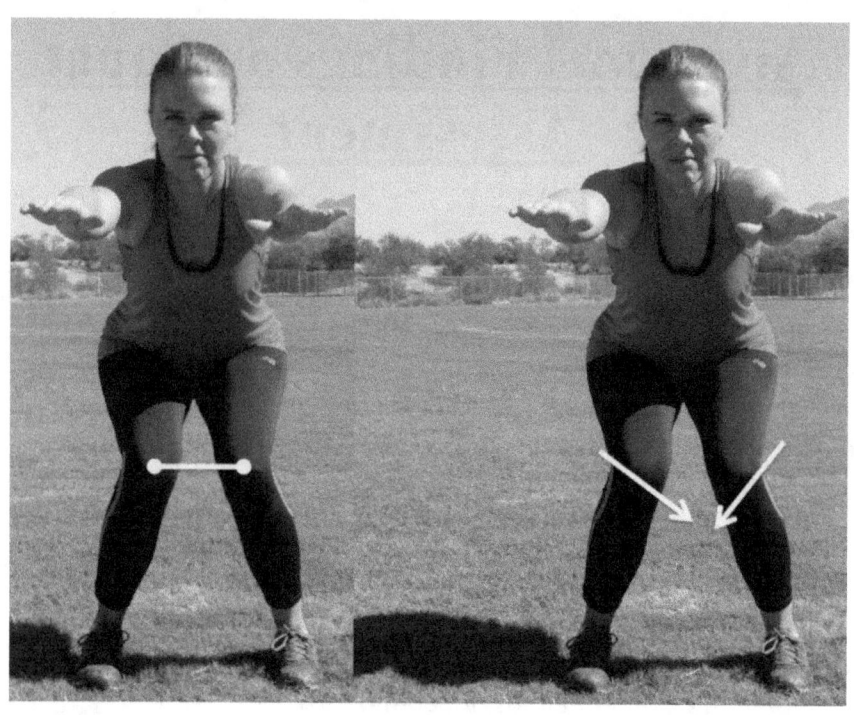

The picture on the following page identifies common problems when looking at the athlete from the side in a squat.

1. The spine is curved and the knees are over the toes.
2. The knees are over the toes. This is a bad position for the knees. It can lead to pain and injury.
3. The head is past the toes. Think about how this moves the center of balance too far forward.
4. Notice that the athlete is looking down towards the ground. This has implications for balance and where the center of gravity is.
5. A significant angle is created at the trunk with the ground. If the trunk is almost parallel with the ground, this is a problem. The appropriate muscle groups will have a very difficult time performing properly in this position.

*** Special Note***

If the athlete is unable to perform a proper squat you may stop the assessment. If the athlete is unable to perform the most basic sport movement, the athlete should be referred to a Physical Therapist for evaluation and initiation of an ACL injury prevention program.

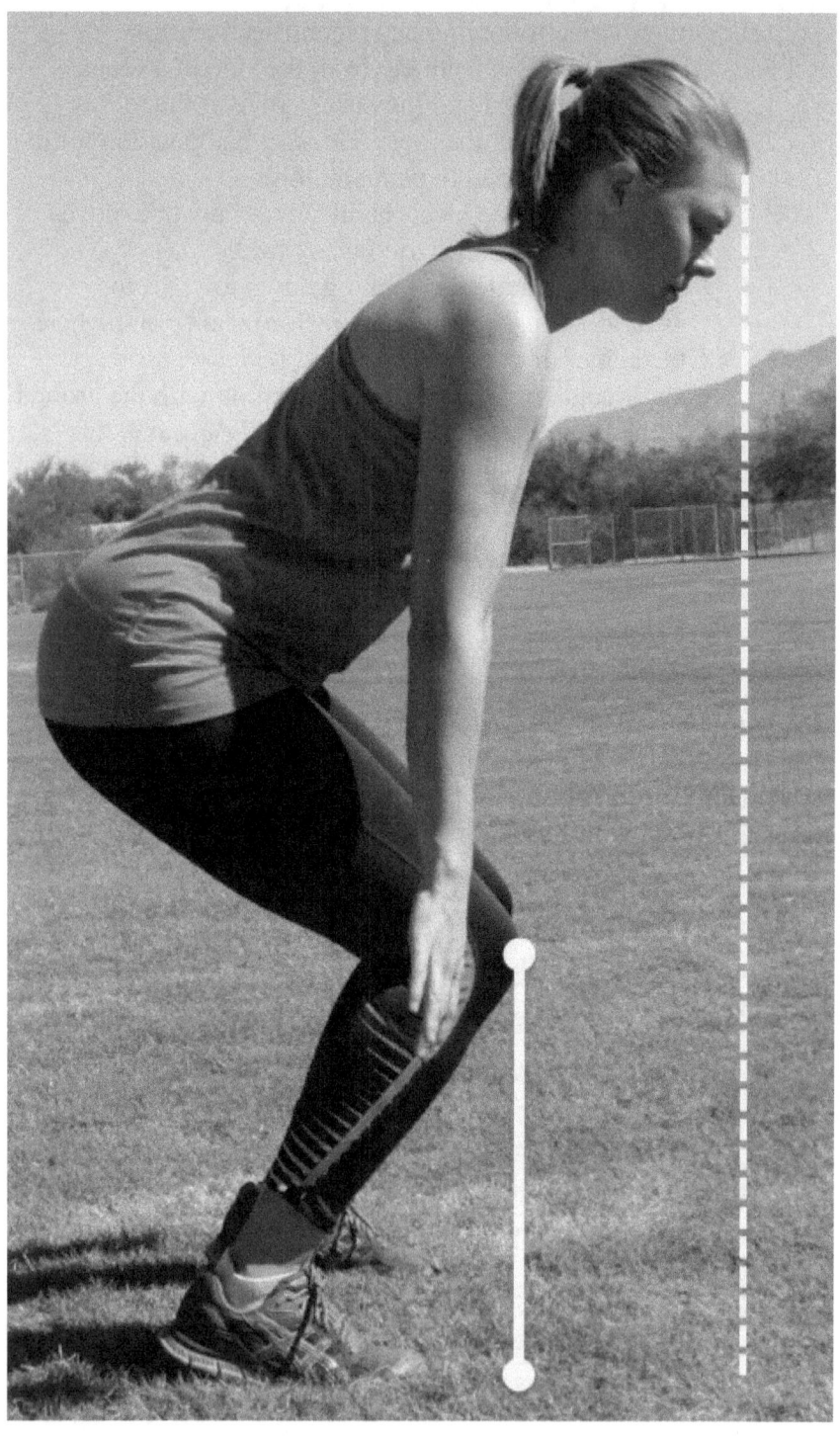

<u>Jump Assessment</u>

If the squats look good, have your athlete jump off of an object 6-18 inches (step, bench, etc). Start on a shorter surface and work your way up. The takeoff and landing should look like the image below.

1. Pay attention to the alignment of the hips, knees, and ankles from the front (should be straight).
2. The arrows identify how the athlete below is able to maintain the knees at shoulder width apart from takeoff to landing which is crucial for safely completing this task. This ability will translate to jumping involved in competition.

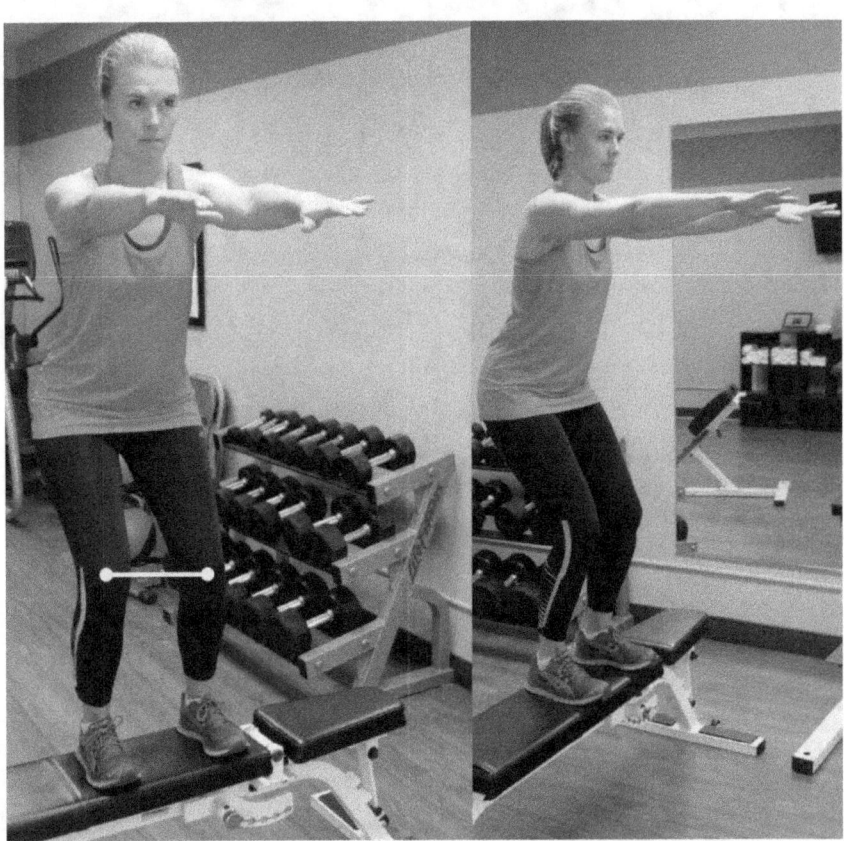

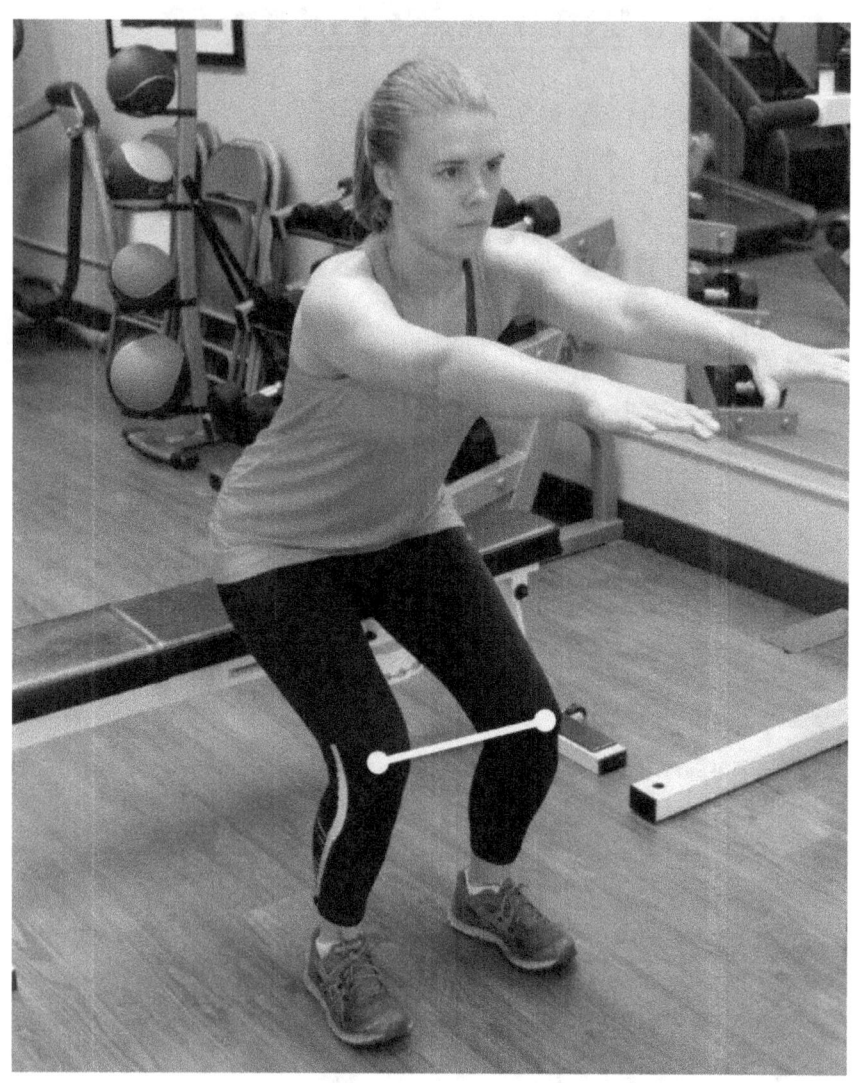

From the side we are able to see a number of things.

1. The knees stay behind the toes from takeoff all the way through landing.
2. The head/neck/spine maintain a straight line.
3. The landing is into a squat position. This should be a smooth landing on the balls of the feet <u>without</u> a loud "thud."
4. The arms rise up to help balance the landing.

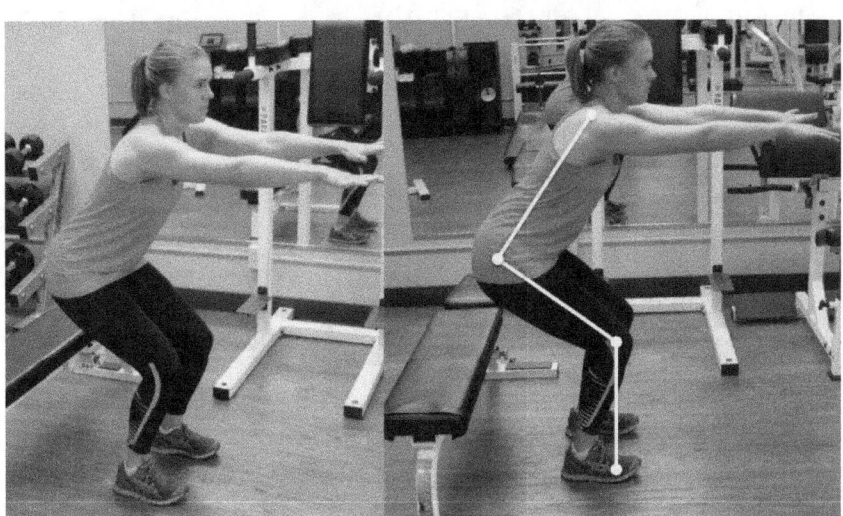

<u>Abnormal Findings on Jump Assessment</u>

The picture below shows someone after jumping off a box and landing. You should be able to draw a straight line through her hip, knee, and ankle. Compare this to the previous picture. In this picture we see:
1. The knees coming forward over the toes.
2. The knees angling in towards the middle.
3. The athlete looking down.
4. Arms remain at the side.

These findings are a recipe for potential disaster.

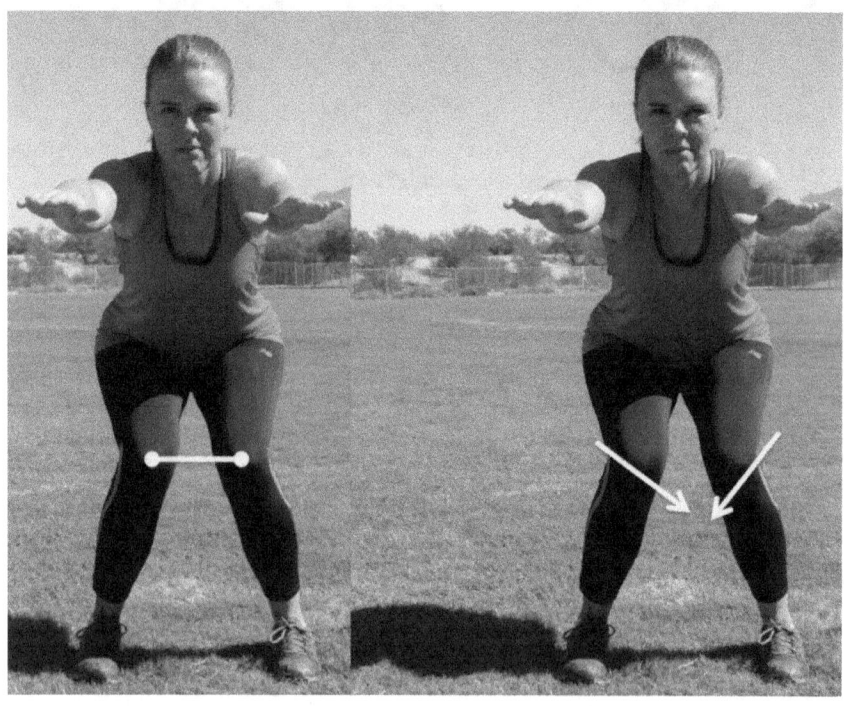

Another sign to watch for is a stiff kneed landing when jumping off the box. Normally, this type of landing is accompanied by a loud "thud." When landing from a jump you want to see the knees and hips bend to absorb the shock. If they land straight legged, this will increase their risk for ACL injury.

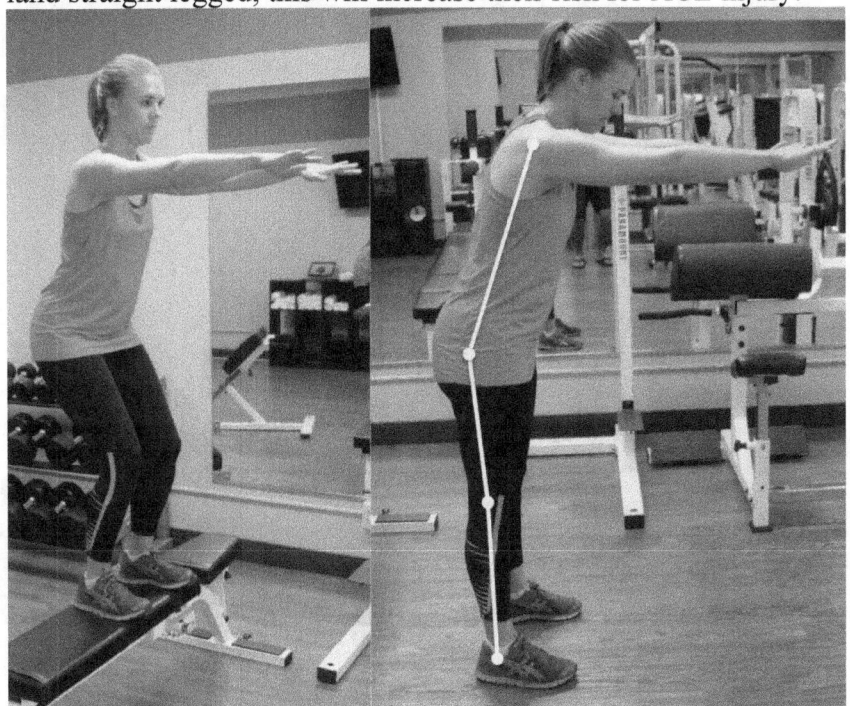

Lunge Assessment

The lunge is up next. It is a more difficult activity in that the feet are moved further apart making maintaining balance more of a challenge. It is also more demanding on strength. If the athlete exhibits balance problems in any of these assessments they are at greater risk of injury. Balance exercises would need to be added to that athlete's strength and conditioning program.

The athlete below is correctly performing the lunge. Note how:

1. The hip/knee/ankle form a straight line (back and front leg).
2. Chest and head are held straight.
3. Arms relaxed at the side.
4. The starting position for a lunge should be standing straight up with one foot well in front of the other- both pointing forward.
5. The athlete should then slowly lower their body down, trunk straight up, weight evenly distributed.
6. Make sure that the back leg is back enough such that in the full lunge the front leg bends to 90 degrees at the knee (with the knee remaining behind the toes).
7. Slowly lower to the ground.
8. The back knee should lightly touch the ground, but not rest upon it.
9. Return to the starting position.
10. The athlete's back should remain straight throughout the lunge.
11. Contracting abdominal muscles helps keep the trunk stable through the lunge.

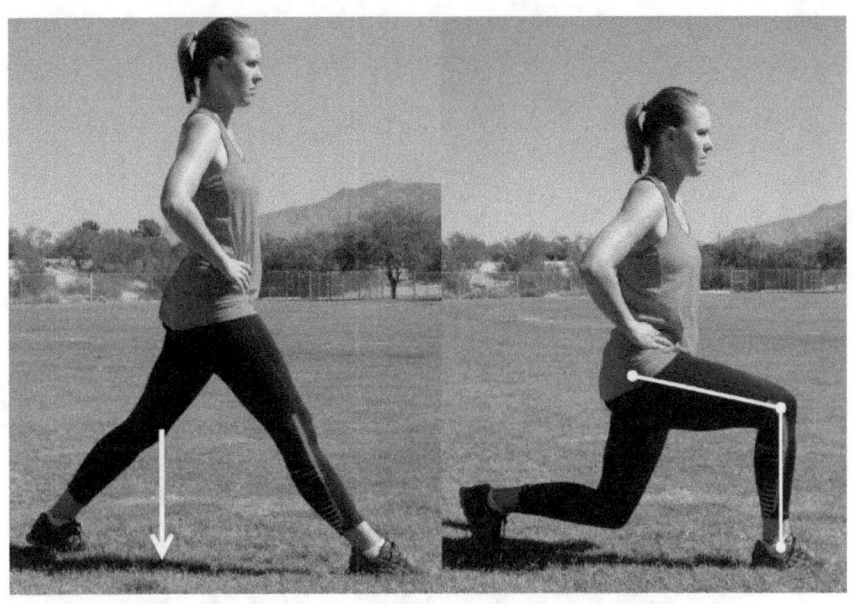

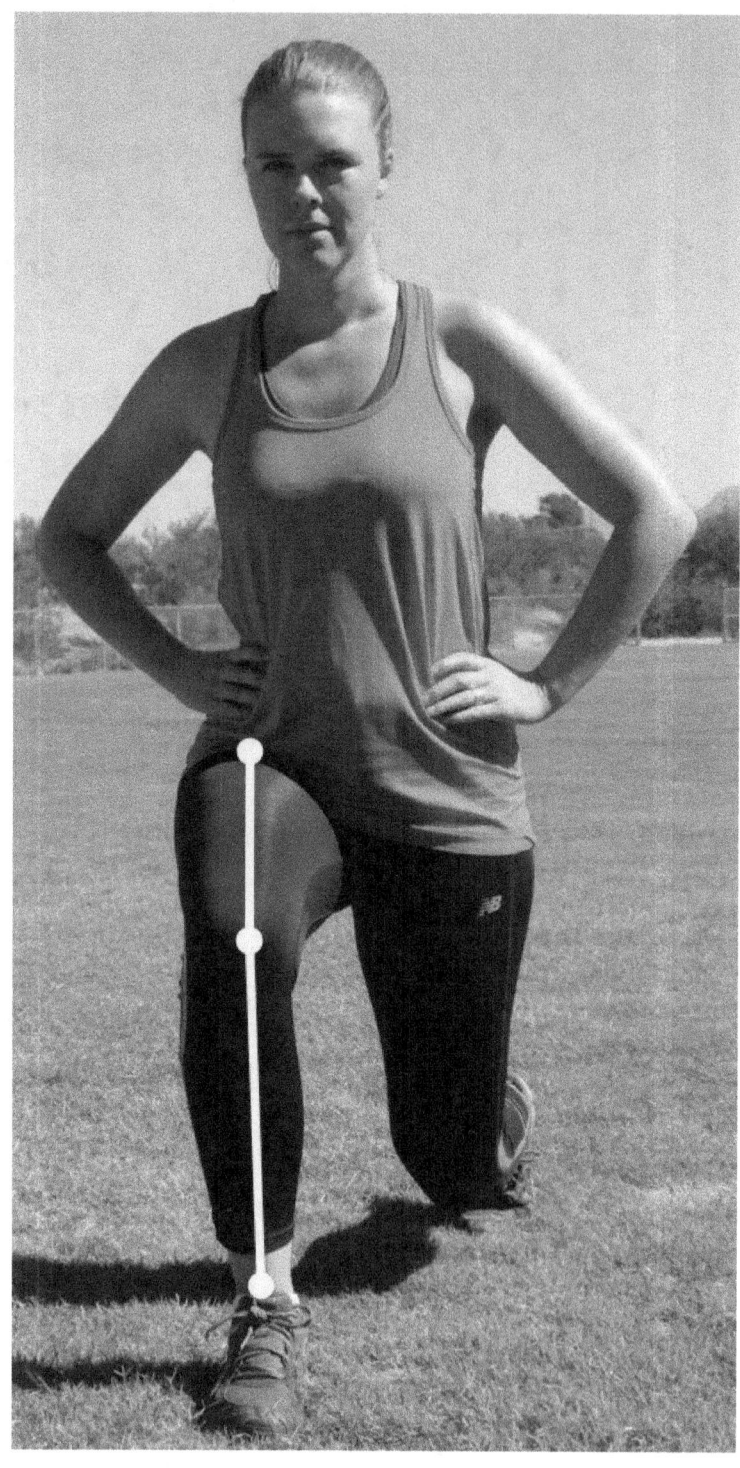

Note how the athlete below is correctly:
1. Creating 90° angles at the hip/knee/ankle of the forward
   leg.
2. Head/neck/chest are straight.

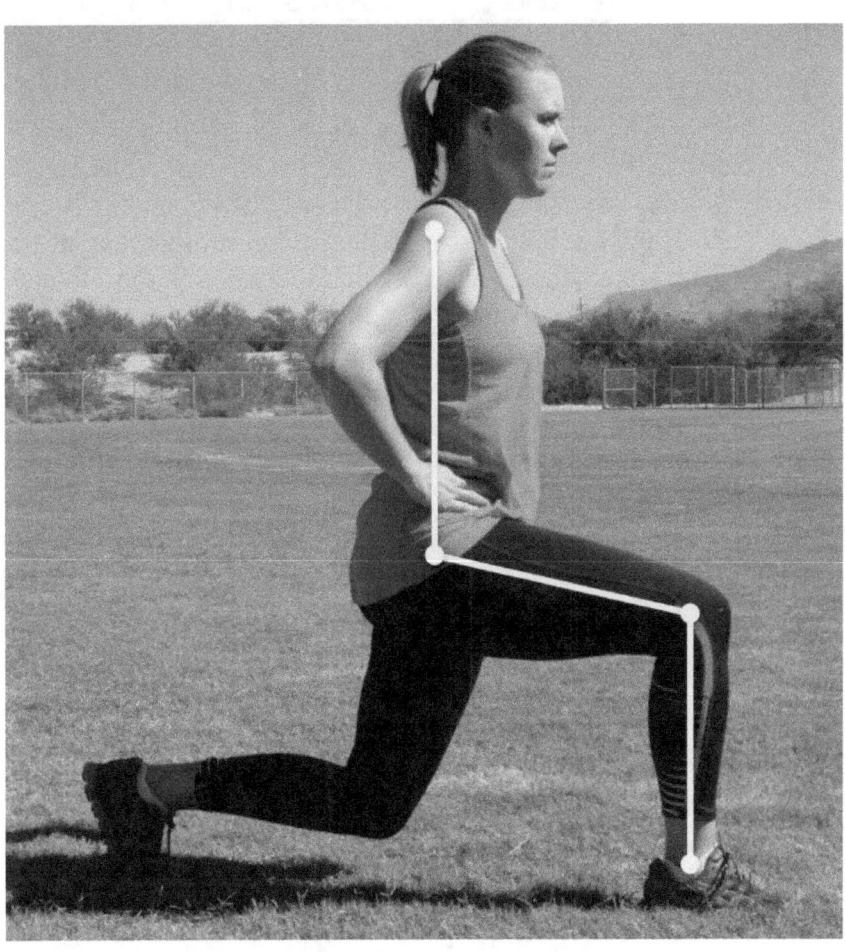

Abnormal Findings on Lunge Assessment

This front view of an athlete is an example of a bad lunge. Notice how the person's knee *crosses the midline* of the body?

1. The hip, knee, and ankle, do not line up.
2. Hip, knee, and ankle should form a straight line, not a crooked one. This is another red flag that this athlete needs to be evaluated and treated.
3. Athletes who lose their balance in a lunge are at increased risk of injury.
4. Athletes who fatigue early in sets of lunges are also at increased risk.

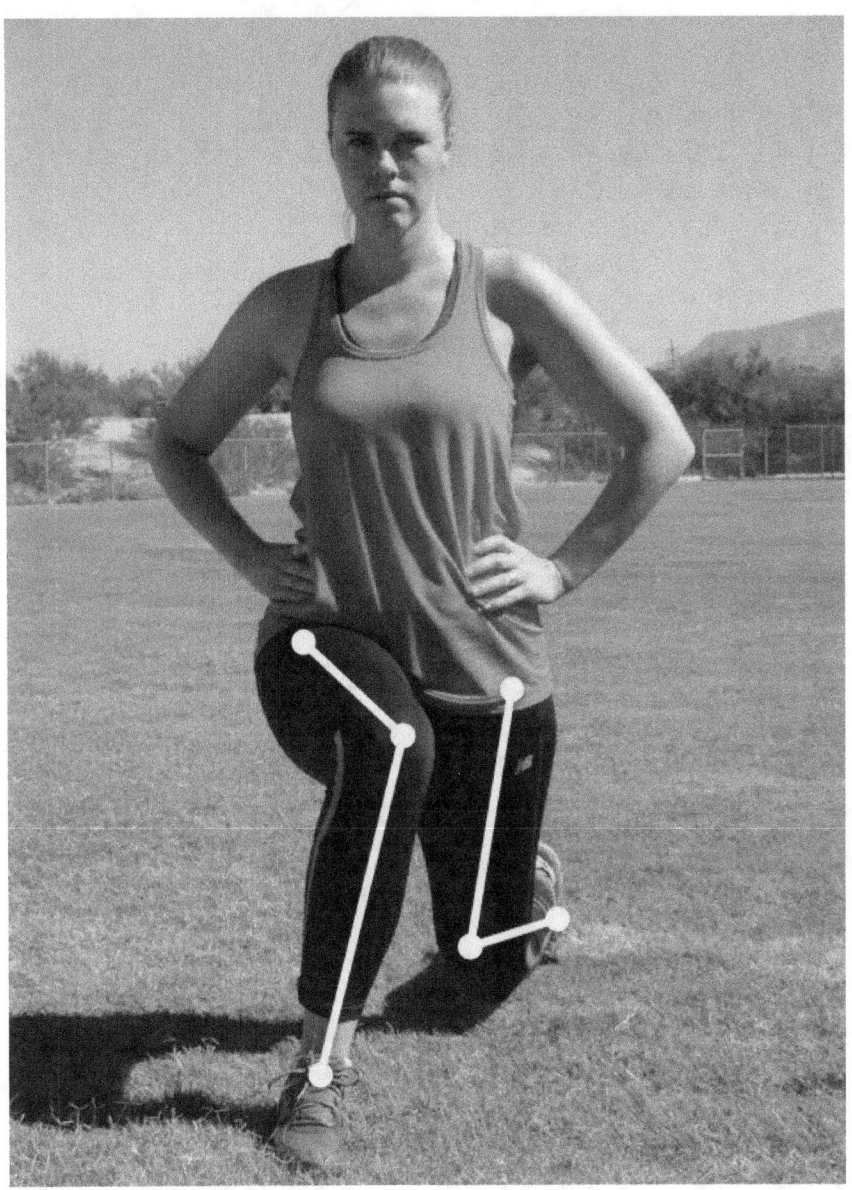

This is a side view of an athlete incorrectly performing the lunge. Note that:
1.   The knee goes over the toes placing unnecessary stress on the knee.
2.   The trunk is pitched forward.
3.   The athlete's upper body is pitched forward.
4.   The back leg is too high off the ground.

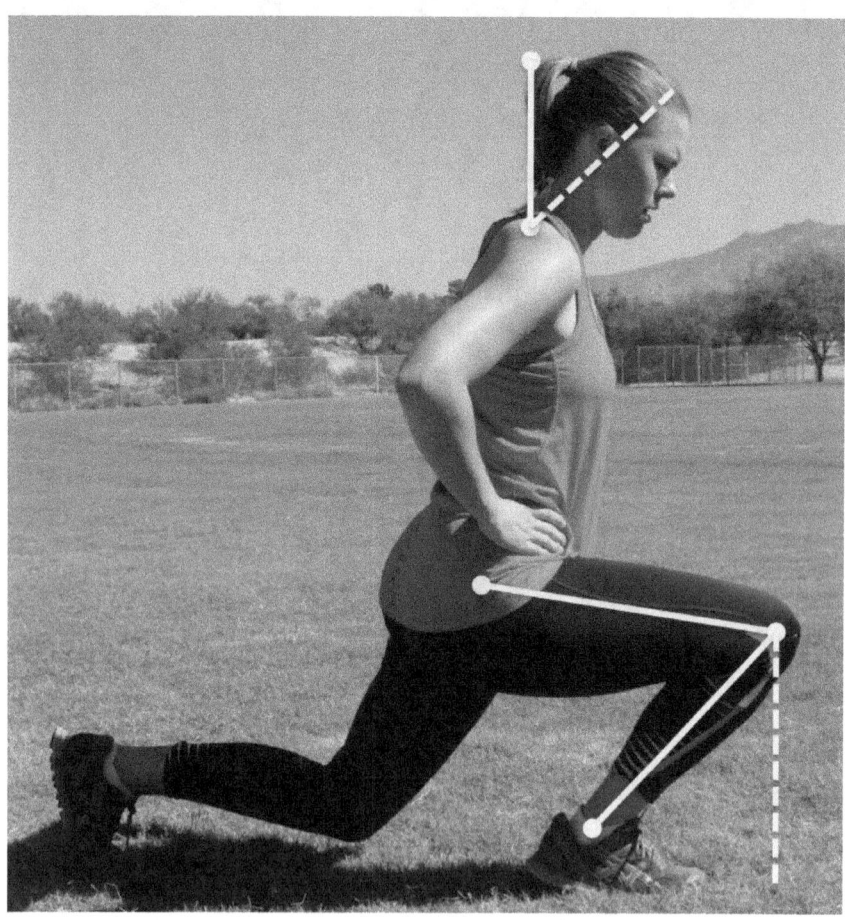

Running Assessment

The final evaluation involves assessing the athlete's mechanics while running. The athlete should run three 40 yard sprints on a field, track, or treadmill (less ideal). They should be observed from behind and from the side.

The images below show proper alignment of hip, knee and foot for a running athlete. Note how a straight line can be drawn from the hip to the ankle. It also shows the runner landing near the rear foot and slightly on the outside of the foot. The back foot is coming off the toes. This is the appropriate landing style during sprinting. Note how the spine is straight and the back hip extends through the running motion.

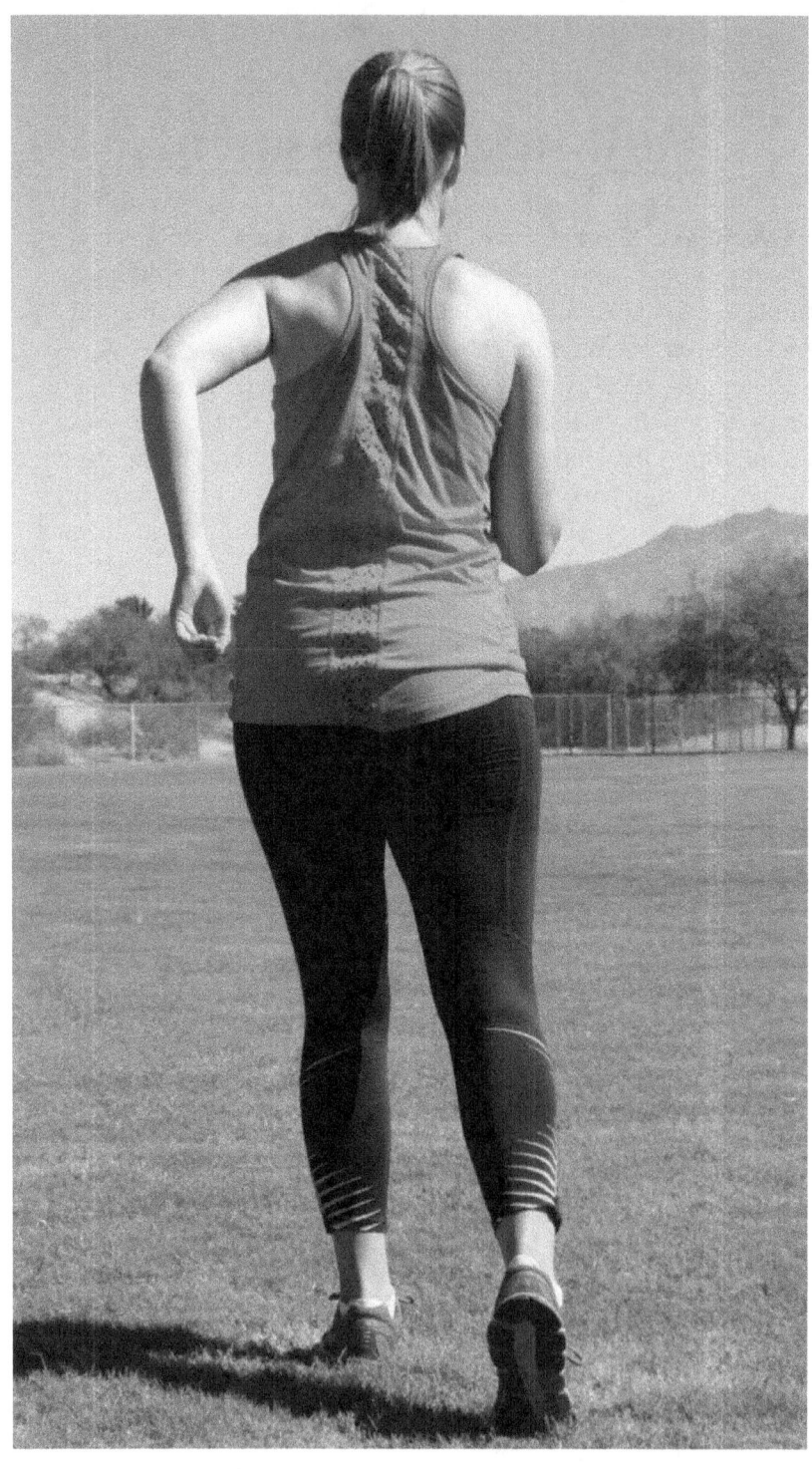

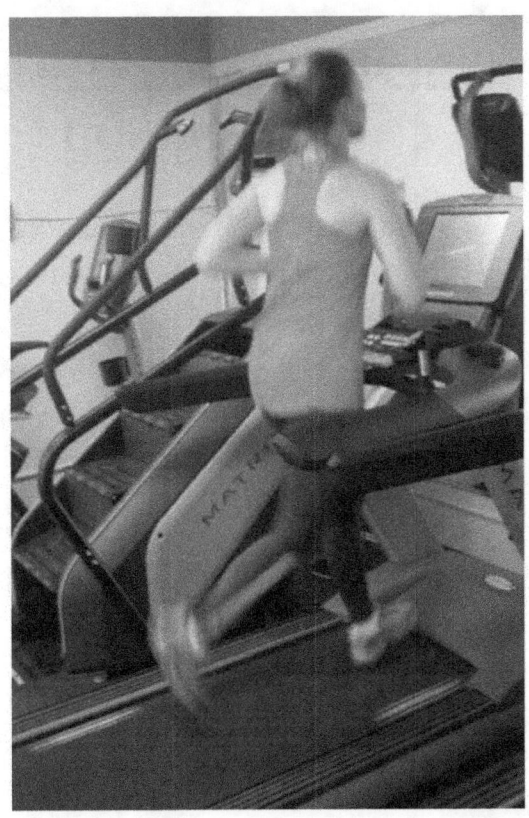

<u>Abnormal Running Assessment</u>

The image below shows you what should <u>NOT</u> be happening during the running assessment.

1. Notice how a line from the hip to the ankle does not go through the knee.
2. Note how the left knee dives in resulting in the left foot to swinging out. If you see this, it is grounds for immediate referral. You would be surprised how often this grossly abnormal motion can be observed in young female athletes!

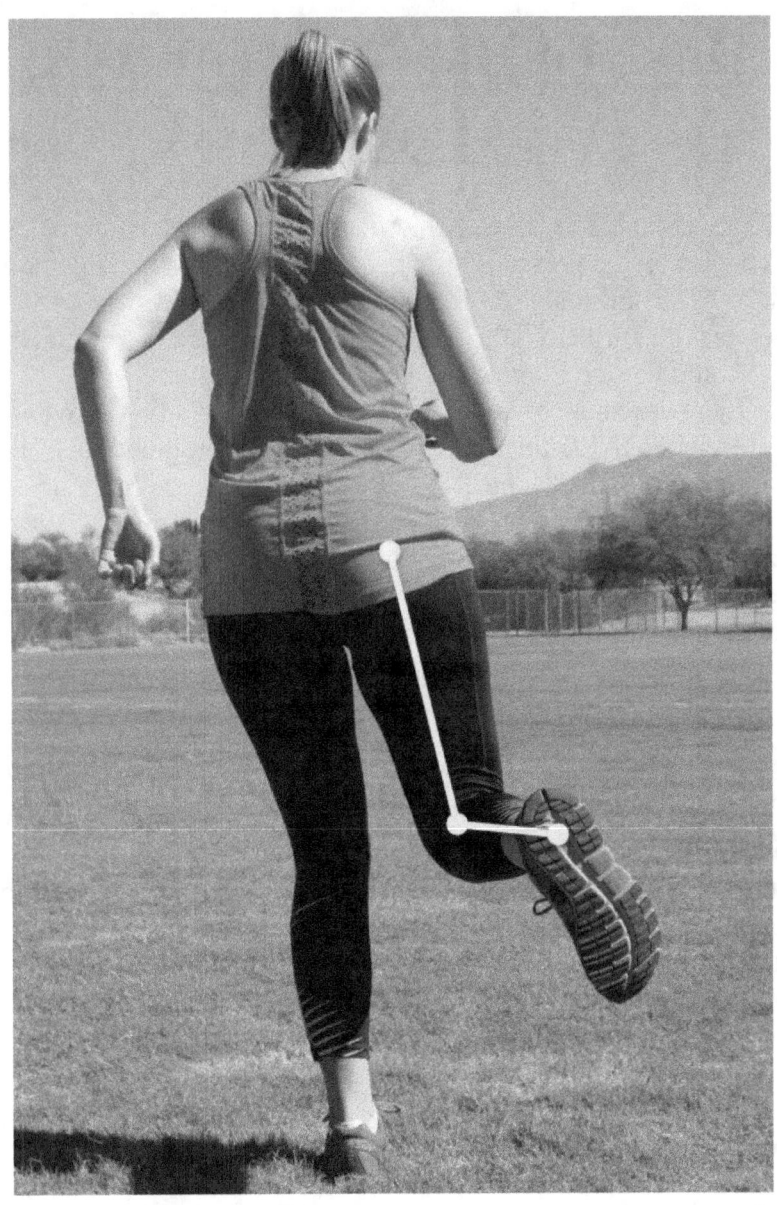

<u>How To Help Prevent ACL Injury</u>

Prevention is the key. Athletes who demonstrate high risk mechanics on the previous tests need to be identified. Athletes at risk of ACL injury ideally should see a qualified Physical Therapist for further evaluation and recommendations. Athletes at risk should be started on an ACL protection program.

There are many great programs out there including Move California, FMARC/the FIFA 11, and the PEP program out of the University of Santa Monica. I have created my own program based on several out there and adjust it to the individual athlete and their sport (see section on my program later). Research has shown that specific ACL injury prevention programs <u>DO</u> work and can significantly reduce the risk of non-contact ACL injuries[5].

The biggest challenge is athlete adherence to the programs. To truly reduce the risk of ACL injuries, most programs call for the exercises to be performed 4+ times per week.

Do not close this book!

I know it is a large commitment, but for the athlete at risk it is well worth it. It takes less time and effort to prevent an ACL injury than it takes to injure an ACL, have surgery, go through the rehabilitation and hope that the athlete will return to her previous performance level.

Where To Start?—The Basics

It amazes me each time an athlete comes in looking to start an ACL program and demands the "high-level exercises" and none of the "simple ones" because they are "an athlete." I start the session by asking: "How many squats can you do?" "Do you do them correctly?" "Really?" "Have you ever had someone take a video of you doing one, or watched yourself in a mirror?"

The vast majority of athletes that come through my door looking to start an ACL injury prevention program cannot perform a single quality squat- with ZERO resistance. I am not kidding!

There are many great programs out there, but the athlete at risk must master the 4 basic exercises outlined in this chapter before she moves on to higher level activities. These exercises are the foundation for everything else the athlete will do in her ACL protection program.

The athlete should perform each exercise demonstrated in this chapter for 3 sets of 10 repetitions. They should take 1 minute breaks in between sets. If the athlete cannot perform these exercises with the proper form, they are not ready to move on!

For videos of the following exercises, please go to:
www.youtube.com/TheSmartLifeSeries
Click on the "**Playlist**" tab and select "**ACL Injury Prevention (Starter)**."

<u>Squats</u>

Muscles Used: glut max, hamstrings, quads

How To: Keep the feet flat on the floor about shoulder width apart with the toes pointing forward. Squat a short distance down leading with your buttocks. The hips lead the movement. Pretend like you are sitting in an invisible chair. Use a chair or countertop for support as needed.

Mistakes: Do NOT let your knees go over your toes. Do NOT let your knees lead the movement.

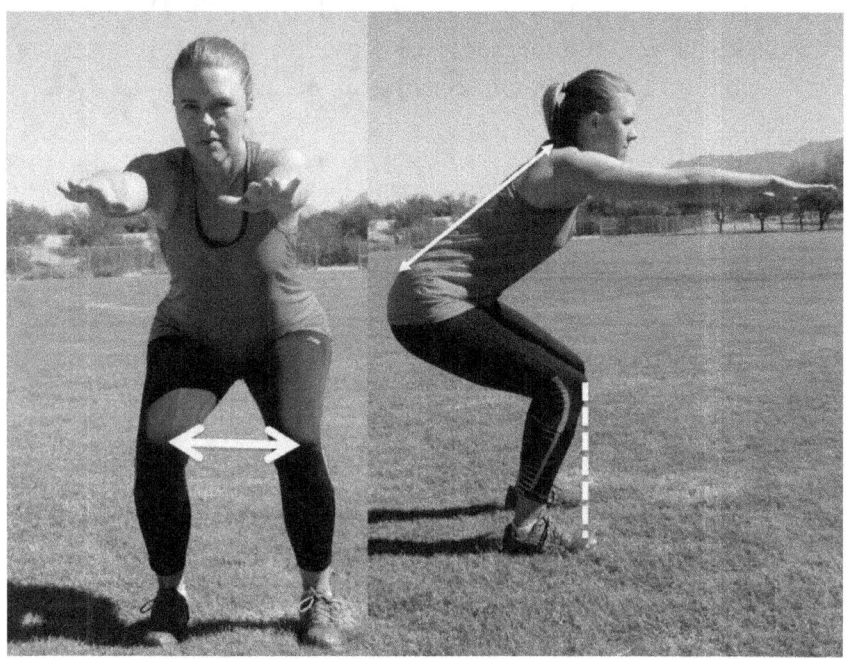

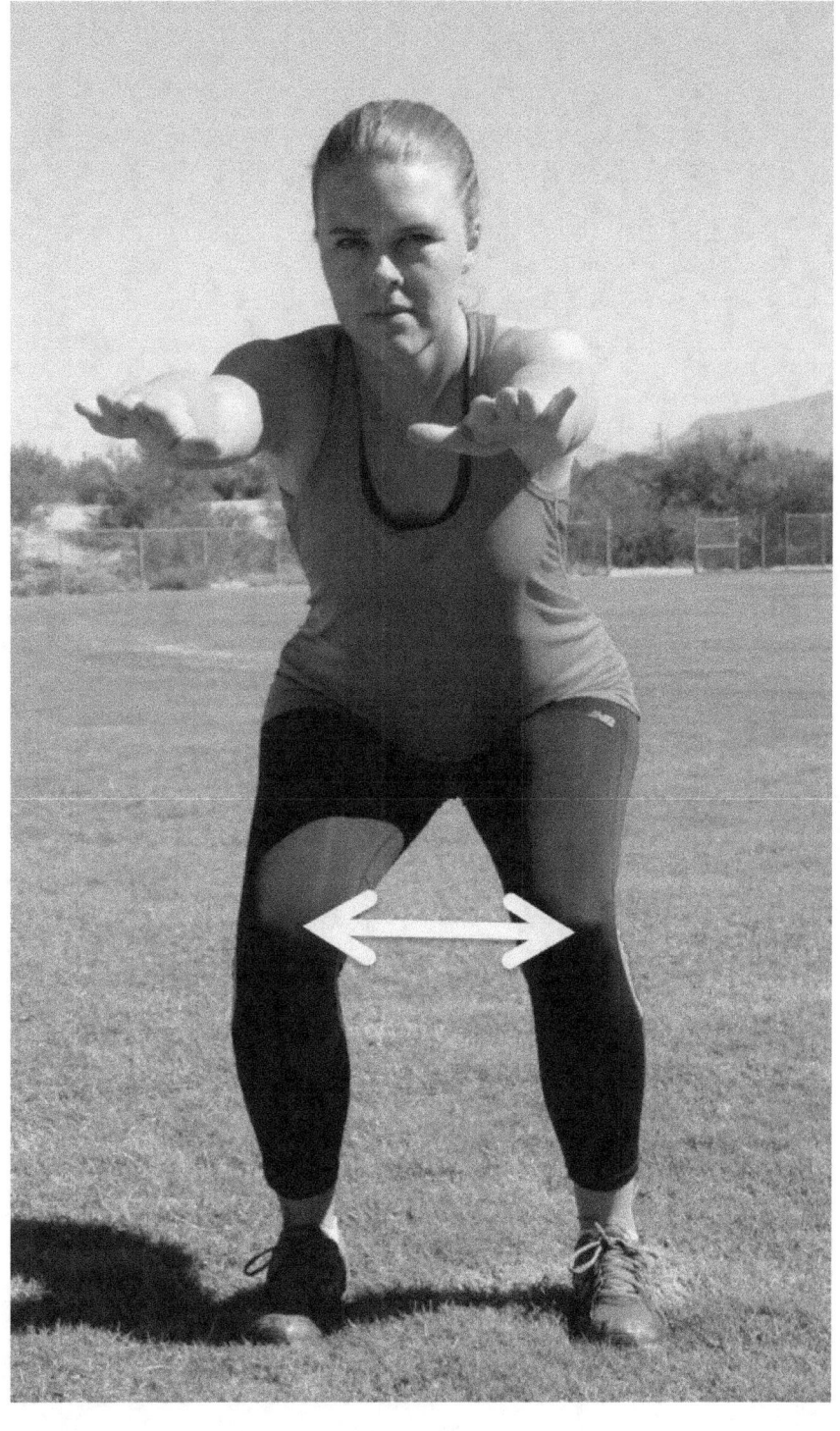

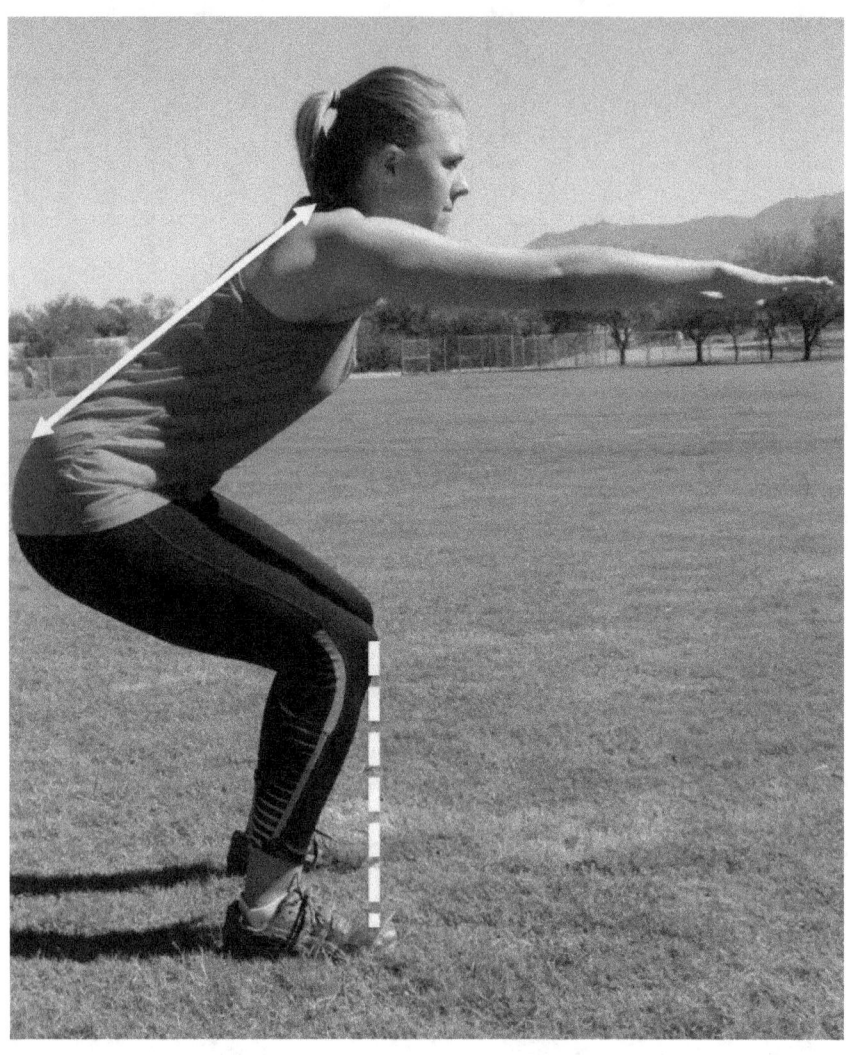

Static Lunges

Muscles Used: quads, glutes

How To: Make sure the back leg is back far enough so that your front leg bends to about 90* without your knee going past your toes. The back knee should lightly touch the ground, but not rest on it. Your back should remain straight at all times without flexing forward. Make sure to engage your abdominals at all times. Stand by a mirror to watch your form.

Mistakes: Your spine should NOT be flexing forward. It should be straight up.

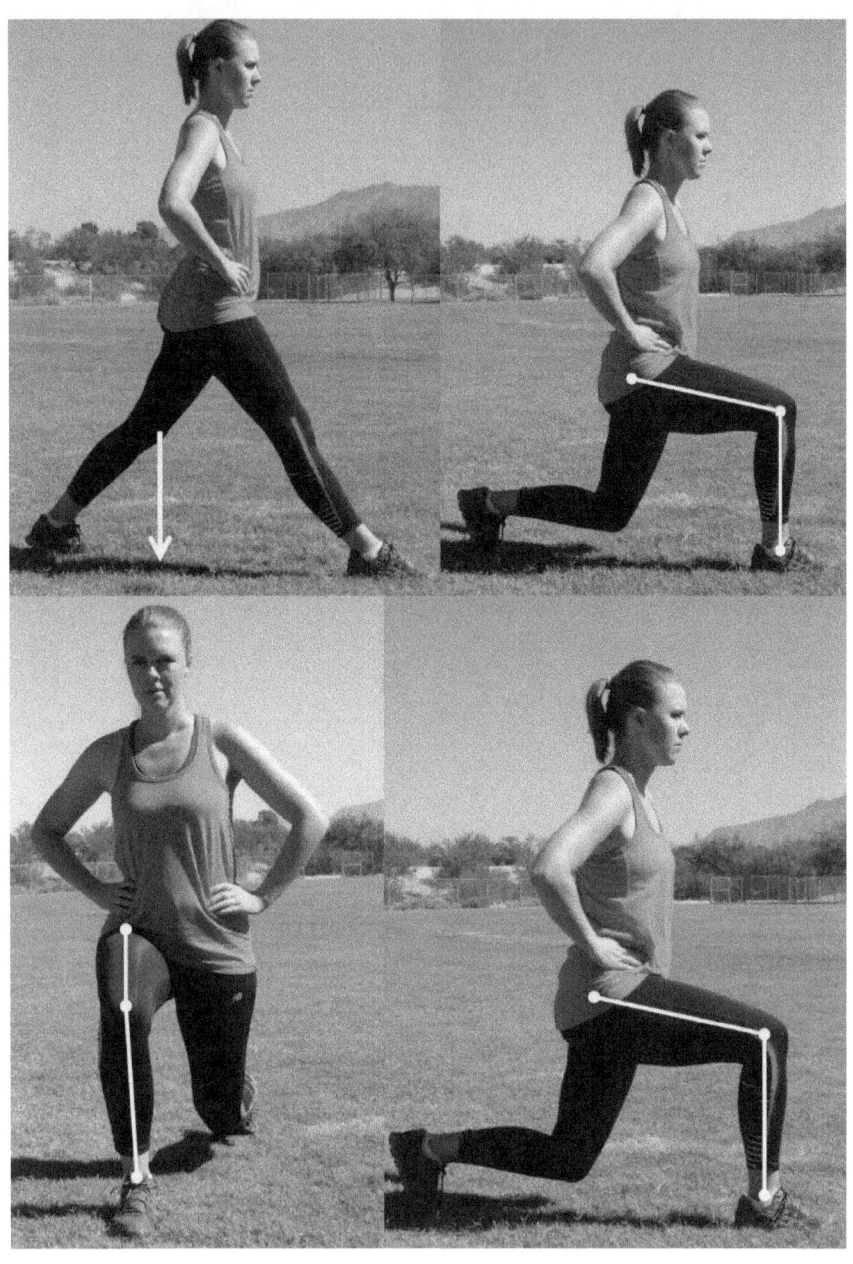

Step Downs

Muscles Used: quads, glutes

How To: Standing on the step, slowly lower the opposite heel to the ground. Pretend as if you are lowering yourself to sit in a chair. Lightly tap the ground with your heel and return to the starting position.

Mistakes: Do NOT let your knee go past your toes as you bend your knee.

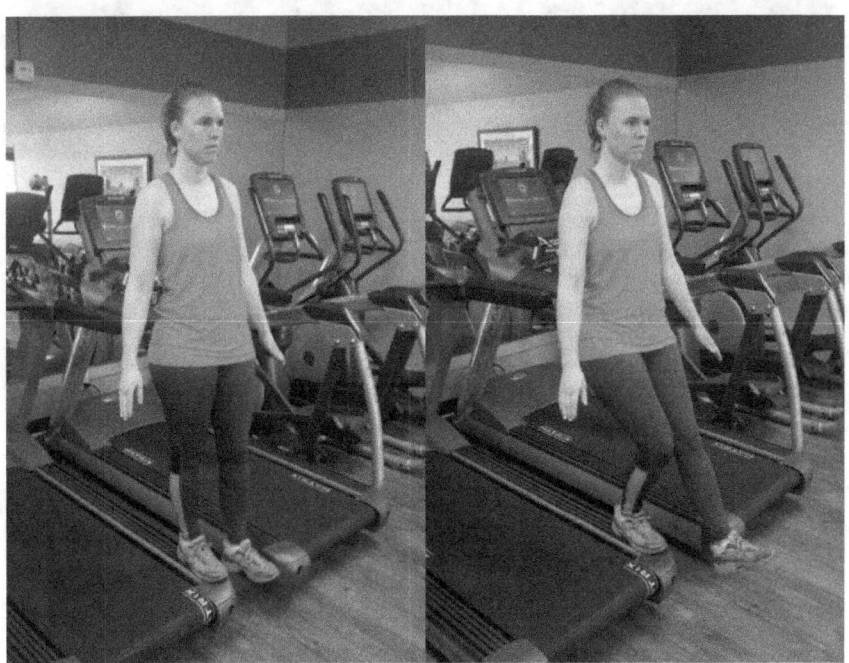

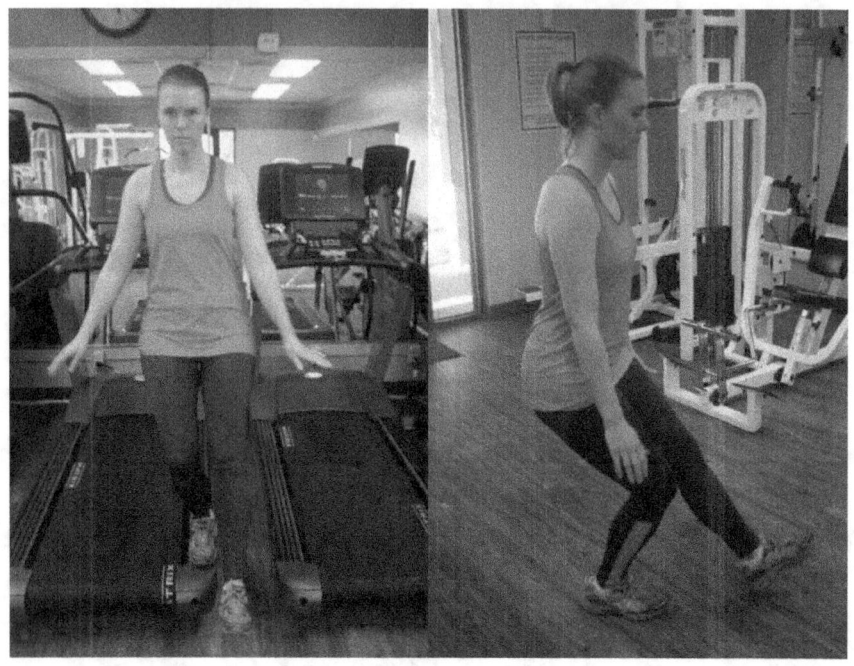

<u>Planks</u>

Muscles Used: abdominals, obliques

How To: Begin on your stomach, with each elbow tucked against your body as pictured. Move as if you were going to do a push up, but only go up onto your elbows. Tailbone should be tucked. Back should be straight. Knees should be off the ground. Chin should be tucked. Keep that tummy tight!

Mistakes: Do NOT arch/hunch your back.

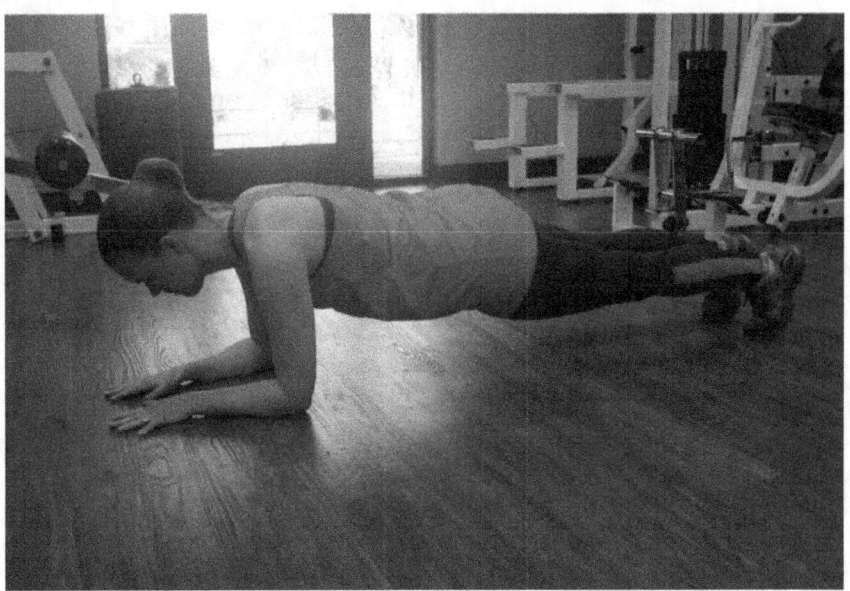

<u>Which Program Is Best For Me?—Advanced Programs</u>

Please note that no advanced programs should be initiated without first consulting a qualified Physical Therapist. Form and technique are EVERYTHING. If the athlete's form is poor, she can perform the exercises every day and not obtain any benefit. Furthermore, if performed incorrectly, the athlete may actually injure themselves.

As far as which program is best for a specific athlete, it is advisable to work this out with a Physical Therapist. Each program has various strengths and weakness. Some will fit better into an athlete's schedule than others. Some will fit the body mechanics of the individual athlete better. Some will fit better the stresses of the athletes individual sport. This is why my program, "The Smart Life ACL Program," incorporates components of multiple programs and adapts to the individual athlete and her needs.

The FMARC–FIFA 11+ (http://f-marc.com/11plus/home/) program is a pre-competition routine using sport specific exercises to prepare the body for the balance and coordination demands of soccer.

Th PEP (http://smsmf.org/smsf-programs/pep-program) program has a large strengthening component. It also includes a static stretching which is not seen in other programs.

<u>My Program (8wks)</u>

The Smart Life ACL Program is a combination of hip/knee strengthening, balance training, plyometrics, and agility training. It is an 8 week program. The program takes place both in the therapy office and at home. The home exercise plan is varied every 2 weeks after assessment by the Physical Therapist. Form is critical- I don't allow ANY cheating! Increasing resistance and difficulty are not engaged unless the athlete's form is correct. Once through the program we strongly encourage the athlete to maintain an appropriate exercise regimen throughout their athletic careers. Multiple ACL risk assessments should be performed throughout the athletes career. For videos of the following exercises, please go to: www.youtube.com/TheSmartLifeSeries Click on the "**Playlist**" tab and select "**ACL Injury Prevention (My Program)**."

<u>Week 1-2</u>
1. Squats
2. Static Lunges
3. Bilateral Heel Raises
4. Plank
5. Side Plank
6. Wall Squats + Band
7. Single Leg Stand With Running Motion
8. Sidelying Hip Abduction
9. Marching Bridges
10. Standing Hamstring Curls

<u>Weeks 3-4</u>
1. Squats

2. Squat Hops
3. Resisted Speed Skaters
4. Unilateral Heel Raise vs. Step
5. Side Lunges
6. Sidelying Hip Abduction
7. Single Leg Stand On Pillow With Running Motion
8. Balance Board/BOSU Ball + Perturbations
9. Bilateral Heel Raise Hops
10. 1-2-3's

Weeks 5-6

1. Monster Walks
2. Heismans
3. Forward/Backwards Running
4. Bounding
5. Cut Off Of Short Step
6. Lunge onto unsteady surface + TB around front knee
7. Single Leg Hop In Place
8. Around The World
9. Balance Board + Perturbations (eyes closed)
10. Squat Hops For Height

Weeks 7-8

1. Depth Jumps
2. Hop Overs Side/Front
3. Scissor Jumps
4. Single Leg Hops Forward/Backward/Diagonal
5. Squat Jump + 180
6. Squat Hops For Height

7. Sprint + Cut
8. Broad Jumps
9. Sprint + Decelerations
10. Sprint + Collisions

Just a reminder that more exercises can be found at:

http://www.youtube.com/TheSmartLifeSeries

AND

http://www.TheSmartLifeSeries.com

<u>References</u>

1. Hewett, TE. Why women have increased risk of ACL injury. American Academy of Orthopedic Surgeons. November 2010
2. Adams, et al. The Effects of Knee Motion and External Loading on the Length of the Anterior Cruciate Ligament (ACL): A Kinematic Study. *J Biomech Eng* 113(2), 208-214 (May 01, 1991) (7 pages)
3. Nilstad, et. al. Physiotherapists can identify female football players with high knee valgus angles during vertical drop jumps using real-time observational screening. Journal of Orthopedic and Sport Physical Therapy. Vol. 44, Issue: 5, Pages: 258-365
4. Tait, et. al. The effects of a home-based instructional program aimed at improving frontal plane knee biomechanics during a jump-landing task. Journal of Orthopedic and Sport Physical Therapy. Vol: 43, Issue: 7, Pages 486-494.
5. Fifa 11+. http://f-marc.com/11plus/home/
6. PEP Program. http://smsmf.org/smsf-programs/pep-program

ABOUT THE AUTHOR

Sean earned his BS in Kinesiology and Exercise Science from James Madison University in 2007. He spent time volunteering in an outpatient physical therapy clinic and in-patient facility with occupational therapy as a student. He completed his Doctorate in Physical Therapy at St. Francis University in 2010 and is a Certified Strength and Conditioning Specialist (CSCS). Last year he completed the certification requirements for Kinesio Taping to become a Certified Kinesio Tape Practitioner (CKTP). Most recently, he participated in the Movement for Life residency in conjunction with the University of Southern California, passed his boards, and is now a Board Certified Orthopedic Clinical Specialist (OCS). He is also a Rock Steady Boxing Coach (a program aimed at helping people with Parkinson's reduce their symptoms). Throughout his schooling he served as a teaching assistant, ran an exercise physiology lab, and enjoyed a unique clinical rotation in the rolling Tuscan hillsides in Italy (improving his Italian language abilities along the way).

After proposing in Scotland, Sean and his soccer star wife have now been married for over 5 years. Sean is an avid sports fan (soccer! and most everything else with a ball), loves traveling the world (Wales is next on his list), speaks Italian, and spends most of his free time with his dogs, on a boat, or in the gym. His hobbies include playing the guitar/mandolin/ukulele, Scottish history, and photography. His areas of interest in physical therapy are sport performance enhancement and orthopedics.

Sean is the creator of a multi-media program *The Smart Life Series* dedicated to helping people develop healthier lifestyles in measured and sustainable ways. The Smart Life Series logo features the silhouette of his brother Colin jumping into the icy waters of February New Hampshire. Check out some of Sean's websites at:
www.TheSmartLifeSeries.com
www.facebook.com/SmartLifeSeries
www.youtube.com/TheSmartLifeSeries

<u>Program Offerings</u>

Sean Simonds is a Doctor of Physical Therapy and Board Certified Orthopedic Clinical Specialist with special interest and expertise in sports performance enhancement. He has helped many women's athletic teams with injury prevention and strength and conditioning programs. He runs "Specialized Physical Therapy of the Carolinas" in Asheville, North Carolina.

He is available at no charge for lectures and seminars on the topic of ACL Injury Prevention as well as many other sports and orthopedic related topics.

He is also available for screening of athletic teams for ACL injury risk. Please contact him at:

Sean@SpecializedNC.com

and the website at: www.SpecializedNC.com

www.ingramcontent.com/pod-product-compliance
Lightning Source LLC
Chambersburg PA
CBHW070440290526
45791CB00005B/2057